DIABETIC COOKBOOKS FOR TYPE 2 DIABETES VEGETARIAN

Plant-Based Meals for Managing Type 2 Diabetes the Delicious Way

T. John

COPYRIGHT PAGE

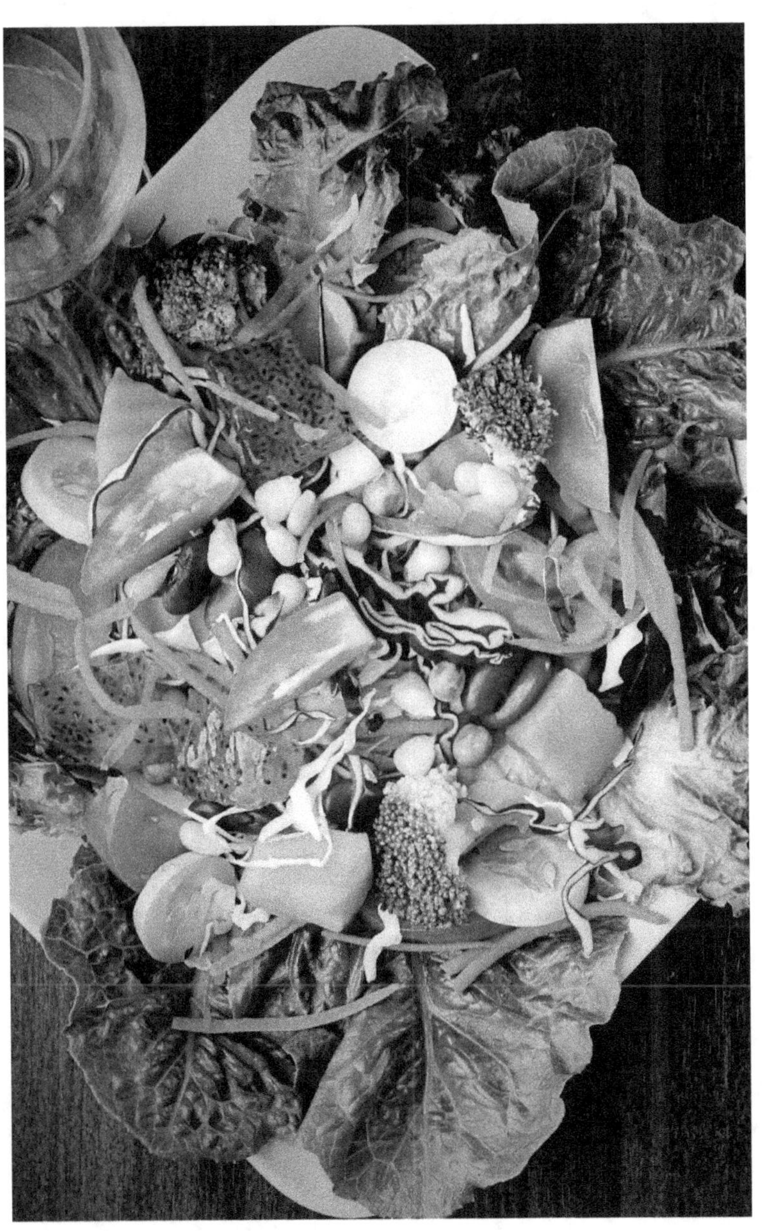

TABLE OF CONTENTS

Chapter 5: Snacks and Appetizers 84

Chapter 6: Desserts 100

Chapter 7: Smoothies 120

INTRODUCTION

Imagine your body as a well-oiled machine. Glucose, the fuel, powers every cog and piston. But in Type 2 diabetes, the gears get a little sticky. Insulin, the key that unlocks the cells for glucose entry, becomes sluggish or scarce. The result? Sugar builds up in the bloodstream, causing a metabolic engine sputter.

Now, picture this: a vibrant kitchen overflowing with kale kaleidoscopes, lentil rainbows, and tofu tangos. This isn't just a culinary scene; it's a potential diabetes management revolution. Enter the vegetarian diet, a plant-based symphony promising to harmonize blood sugar and overall health.

But hold on, veggie-curious souls! Before diving headfirst into bean burgers and chickpea curries, let's unpack the science behind this dietary melody. The magic lies in the fiber fiesta. Unlike their refined counterparts, whole grains, legumes, and vegetables waltz into your gut with a fiber entourage. This fibrous posse slows down glucose absorption, preventing blood sugar spikes and dips. It's like a built-in dimmer switch for your metabolic engine.

But the benefits go beyond a mere blood sugar smoothening. Vegetarian diets tend to be lower in saturated fat and cholesterol, the villainous duo lurking in fatty meats. This translates to reduced risk of heart disease, a frequent diabetes co-star. Plus, the antioxidant orchestra conducted by colorful fruits and vegetables helps keep inflammation at bay, another bonus for overall well-being.

Okay, convinced? Vegetarianism sounds like a diabetes management dream team. But wait, there's a plot twist! Not all plant-based diets are created equal. Sugar masquerading as fruit juices, calorie-dense fried tofu nuggets, and refined carbs disguised as veggie burgers can still throw your blood sugar out of whack. The key is to embrace the whole-food symphony, opting for unprocessed, vibrantly colored ingredients as your lead singers.

Remember, transitioning to a new dietary paradigm is a marathon, not a sprint. Start by incorporating small, plant-powered swaps into your daily routine. Swap that sugary cereal for a nut-and-berry muesli, replace evening takeout with a lentil-bolognese bonanza, and snack on roasted chickpeas instead of cookies. Listen to your body, experiment with flavors, and find joy in the culinary journey.

Most importantly, remember, you're not alone in this veggie tango. Consult a registered dietitian or diabetes educator for personalized guidance. They can help you craft a plant-based melody that harmonizes with your unique needs and preferences.

So, dear reader, embrace the vibrant potential of a vegetarian diet. It's not just about swapping plates; it's about rewriting your diabetes story with each delicious, plant-powered bite. Remember, even the mightiest engines run smoothly with the right fuel. Choose carrots over casseroles, and let your health sing a symphony of well-being.

Chapter 1: 30-Day Meal Plan

Week 1:

Day 1:

- Breakfast: Quinoa and Berry Breakfast Bowl
- Lunch: Lentil and Vegetable Soup
- Dinner: Baked Eggplant Parmesan
- Snack: Guacamole with Vegetable Sticks
- Dessert: Berry and Almond Crisp

Day 2:

- Breakfast: Spinach and Feta Omelette
- Lunch: Quinoa Salad with Roasted Vegetables
- Dinner: Cauliflower Fried Rice with Tofu
- Snack: Baked Sweet Potato Fries
- Dessert: Dark Chocolate Avocado Mousse

Day 3:

- Breakfast: Avocado Toast with Cherry Tomatoes
- Lunch: Chickpea and Spinach Stuffed Bell Peppers

- Dinner: Stuffed Bell Peppers with Quinoa and Black Beans
- Snack: Hummus and Whole Grain Crackers
- Dessert: Coconut Chia Seed Pudding

Day 4:

- Breakfast: Chia Seed Pudding with Almond Milk
- Lunch: Zucchini Noodles with Pesto and Cherry Tomatoes
- Dinner: Spaghetti Squash Primavera
- Snack: Greek Yogurt and Berry Popsicles
- Dessert: Baked Apple with Cinnamon

Day 5:

- Breakfast: Vegetable and Tofu Scramble
- Lunch: Brown Rice and Black Bean Burrito Bowl
- Dinner: Mushroom and Lentil Shepherd's Pie
- Snack: Edamame and Sea Salt
- Dessert: Vegan Chocolate Chip Cookies

Day 6:

- Breakfast: Greek Yogurt Parfait with Nuts and Berries
- Lunch: Caprese Salad with Balsamic Glaze
- Dinner: Tofu and Vegetable Stir-Fry
- Snack: Roasted Chickpeas with Paprika
- Dessert: Almond Flour Banana Bread

Day 7:

- Breakfast: Sweet Potato and Black Bean Breakfast Burrito
- Lunch: Grilled Eggplant and Hummus Wrap
- Dinner: Sweet Potato and Kale Gnocchi
- Snack: Avocado Salsa with Whole Grain Tortilla Chips
- Dessert: Strawberry Shortcake with Almond Flour Biscuits

Week 2:

Day 8:

- Breakfast: Whole Wheat Pancakes with Sugar-Free Syrup

- Lunch: Cauliflower and Broccoli Quiche

- Dinner: Vegan Chili with Kidney Beans

- Snack: Cucumber Rolls with Herbed Cream Cheese

- Dessert: Pistachio and Raspberry Energy Bites

Day 9:

- Breakfast: Berry and Almond Smoothie Bowl

- Lunch: Cucumber and Avocado Sushi Rolls

- Dinner: Portobello Mushroom Fajitas

- Snack: Nut Mix with Dried Fruits

- Dessert: Blueberry and Lemon Frozen Yogurt

Day 10:

- Breakfast: Overnight Oats with Cinnamon and Apples

- Lunch: Sweet Potato and Chickpea Curry

- Dinner: Lemon Garlic Asparagus and Quinoa

- Snack: Stuffed Mushrooms with Spinach and Feta

- Dessert: Pumpkin Pie Smoothie Bowl

Day 11:

- Breakfast: Vegetable and Cheese Breakfast Quesadilla
- Lunch: Mediterranean Chickpea Salad
- Dinner: Ratatouille with Herbed Polenta
- Snack: Caprese Skewers with Balsamic Glaze
- Dessert: Avocado Lime Cheesecake

Day 12:

- Breakfast: Pumpkin and Walnut Muffins
- Lunch: Spinach and Mushroom Quesadilla
- Dinner: Lentil and Vegetable Curry
- Snack: Beet and Goat Cheese Crostini
- Dessert: Chocolate Covered Strawberries

Day 13:

- Breakfast: Blueberry Almond Baked Oatmeal
- Lunch: Tomato Basil Bruschetta
- Dinner: Stuffed Acorn Squash with Wild Rice
- Snack: Apple Slices with Almond Butter
- Dessert: Raspberry Almond Tart

Day 14:

- Breakfast: Broccoli and Cheese Mini Frittatas
- Lunch: Roasted Vegetable and Quinoa Stuffed Portobello Mushrooms
- Dinner: Brussels Sprouts and Pecan Salad
- Snack: Kale Chips with Nutritional Yeast
- Dessert: Mango Sorbet with Mint

Week 3:

Day 15:

- Breakfast: Almond Butter and Banana Sandwich
- Lunch: Black Bean and Corn Quesadilla
- Dinner: Butternut Squash and Sage Risotto
- Snack: Mango and Black Bean Salsa
- Dessert: Vanilla Bean Coconut Rice Pudding

Day 16:

- Breakfast: Quinoa and Berry Breakfast Bowl
- Lunch: Lentil and Vegetable Soup
- Dinner: Baked Eggplant Parmesan
- Snack: Guacamole with Vegetable Sticks
- Dessert: Berry and Almond Crisp

Day 17:

- Breakfast: Spinach and Feta Omelette
- Lunch: Quinoa Salad with Roasted Vegetables
- Dinner: Cauliflower Fried Rice with Tofu
- Snack: Baked Sweet Potato Fries
- Dessert: Dark Chocolate Avocado Mousse

Day 18:

- Breakfast: Avocado Toast with Cherry Tomatoes
- Lunch: Chickpea and Spinach Stuffed Bell Peppers
- Dinner: Stuffed Bell Peppers with Quinoa and Black Beans
- Snack: Hummus and Whole Grain Crackers
- Dessert: Coconut Chia Seed Pudding

Day 19:

- Breakfast: Chia Seed Pudding with Almond Milk
- Lunch: Zucchini Noodles with Pesto and Cherry Tomatoes
- Dinner: Spaghetti Squash Primavera
- Snack: Greek Yogurt and Berry Popsicles
- Dessert: Baked Apple with Cinnamon

Day 20:

- Breakfast: Vegetable and Tofu Scramble
- Lunch: Brown Rice and Black Bean Burrito Bowl
- Dinner: Mushroom and Lentil Shepherd's Pie
- Snack: Edamame and Sea Salt
- Dessert: Vegan Chocolate Chip Cookies

Day 21:

- Breakfast: Greek Yogurt Parfait with Nuts and Berries
- Lunch: Caprese Salad with Balsamic Glaze
- Dinner: Tofu and Vegetable Stir-Fry
- Snack: Roasted Chickpeas with Paprika
- Dessert: Almond Flour Banana Bread

Week 4:

Day 22:

- Breakfast: Sweet Potato and Black Bean Breakfast Burrito
- Lunch: Grilled Eggplant and Hummus Wrap
- Dinner: Sweet Potato and Kale Gnocchi

- Snack: Avocado Salsa with Whole Grain Tortilla
  Chips
- Dessert: Strawberry Shortcake with Almond Flour
  Biscuits

Day 23:

- Breakfast: Whole Wheat Pancakes with Sugar-Free
  Syrup
- Lunch: Cauliflower and Broccoli Quiche
- Dinner: Vegan Chili with Kidney Beans
- Snack: Cucumber Rolls with Herbed Cream Cheese
- Dessert: Pistachio and Raspberry Energy Bites

Day 24:

- Breakfast: Berry and Almond Smoothie Bowl
- Lunch: Cucumber and Avocado Sushi Rolls
- Dinner: Portobello Mushroom Fajitas
- Snack: Nut Mix with Dried Fruits
- Dessert: Blueberry and Lemon Frozen Yogurt

Day 25:

- Breakfast: Overnight Oats with Cinnamon and Apples
- Lunch: Sweet Potato and Chickpea Curry
- Dinner: Lemon Garlic Asparagus and Quinoa
- Snack: Stuffed Mushrooms with Spinach and Feta
- Dessert: Pumpkin Pie Smoothie Bowl

Day 26:

- Breakfast: Vegetable and Cheese Breakfast Quesadilla
- Lunch: Mediterranean Chickpea Salad
- Dinner: Ratatouille with Herbed Polenta
- Snack: Caprese Skewers with Balsamic Glaze
- Dessert: Avocado Lime Cheesecake

Day 27:

- Breakfast: Pumpkin and Walnut Muffins
- Lunch: Spinach and Mushroom Quesadilla
- Dinner: Lentil and Vegetable Curry
- Snack: Beet and Goat Cheese Crostini
- Dessert: Chocolate Covered Strawberries

Day 28:

- Breakfast: Blueberry Almond Baked Oatmeal
- Lunch: Tomato Basil Bruschetta
- Dinner: Stuffed Acorn Squash with Wild Rice
- Snack: Apple Slices with Almond Butter
- Dessert: Raspberry Almond Tart

Day 29:

- Breakfast: Broccoli and Cheese Mini Frittatas
- Lunch: Roasted Vegetable and Quinoa Stuffed Portobello Mushrooms
- Dinner: Brussels Sprouts and Pecan Salad
- Snack: Kale Chips with Nutritional Yeast
- Dessert: Mango Sorbet with Mint

Day 30:

- Breakfast: Almond Butter and Banana Sandwich
- Lunch: Black Bean and Corn Quesadilla
- Dinner: Butternut Squash and Sage Risotto
- Snack: Mango and Black Bean Salsa
- Dessert: Vanilla Bean Coconut Rice Pudding

Chapter 2: Breakfast Recipes

In this chapter, we've curated a collection of vibrant and satisfying breakfast recipes tailored for those managing type 2 diabetes through a vegetarian lifestyle.

Quinoa and Berry Breakfast Bowl

Ingredients:

- 1/2 cup quinoa, rinsed
- 1 cup mixed berries (strawberries, blueberries, raspberries)
- 1 tablespoon chopped nuts (almonds or walnuts)
- 1 tablespoon honey or maple syrup
- 1/2 teaspoon vanilla extract
- 1/2 cup Greek yogurt

Instructions:

1. Cook quinoa according to package instructions and let it cool.

2. In a bowl, combine cooked quinoa, mixed berries, chopped nuts, honey or maple syrup, and vanilla extract.

3. Top with Greek yogurt and enjoy!

Nutrition Information (per serving):

- Calories: 300
- Protein: 10g
- Carbohydrates: 45g
- Fat: 8g
- Fiber: 6g
- Sugar: 15g
- Portion Size: 1 serving

Spinach and Feta Omelette

Ingredients:

- 2 large eggs
- 1 cup fresh spinach, chopped
- 2 tablespoons crumbled feta cheese
- 1 tablespoon olive oil
- Salt and pepper to taste

Instructions:

1. Whisk eggs in a bowl and season with salt and pepper.
2. Heat olive oil in a pan over medium heat, add spinach, and sauté until wilted.
3. Pour whisked eggs over spinach, sprinkle feta cheese, and cook until set.
4. Fold the omelette in half, slide it onto a plate, and serve.

Nutrition Information (per serving):

*   Calories: 250
*   Protein: 15g
*   Carbohydrates: 3g
*   Fat: 18g
*   Fiber: 1g
*   Sugar: 1g
*   Portion Size: 1 serving

Avocado Toast with Cherry Tomatoes

Ingredients:

- 1 slice whole-grain bread
- 1/2 ripe avocado
- 1/2 cup cherry tomatoes, halved
- Salt, pepper, and red pepper flakes to taste
- Fresh basil leaves for garnish

Instructions:

1. Toast the whole-grain bread to your liking.
2. Mash the ripe avocado and spread it on the toasted bread.
3. Top with cherry tomatoes, season with salt, pepper, and red pepper flakes.
4. Garnish with fresh basil leaves and enjoy!

Nutrition Information (per serving):

- Calories: 200
- Protein: 4g
- Carbohydrates: 20g
- Fat: 12g

- Fiber: 7g

- Sugar: 2g

- Portion Size: 1 serving

Chia Seed Pudding with Almond Milk

Ingredients:

- 3 tablespoons chia seeds

- 1 cup unsweetened almond milk

- 1/2 teaspoon vanilla extract

- 1 tablespoon maple syrup or sweetener of choice

- Fresh berries for topping

Instructions:

1. In a bowl, mix chia seeds, almond milk, vanilla extract, and maple syrup.

2. Stir well and refrigerate for at least 2 hours or overnight.

3. Before serving, stir the pudding and top with fresh berries.

Nutrition Information (per serving):

- Calories: 150

- Protein: 4g

- Carbohydrates: 18g

- Fat: 8g

- Fiber: 8g

- Sugar: 6g

- Portion Size: 1 serving

Vegetable and Tofu Scramble

Ingredients:

- 1/2 cup firm tofu, crumbled

- 1/2 cup bell peppers, diced

- 1/2 cup cherry tomatoes, halved

- 1/4 cup red onion, chopped

- 1 tablespoon olive oil

- 1/2 teaspoon turmeric powder

- Salt and pepper to taste

Instructions:

1. Heat olive oil in a pan, add red onion, bell peppers, and cherry tomatoes. Sauté until tender.

2. Add crumbled tofu, turmeric powder, salt, and pepper. Cook until tofu is heated through.

3. Serve hot and enjoy a flavorful tofu scramble.

Nutrition Information (per serving):

- Calories: 220
- Protein: 12g
- Carbohydrates: 10g
- Fat: 15g
- Fiber: 3g
- Sugar: 4g
- Portion Size: 1 serving

Greek Yogurt Parfait with Nuts and Berries

Ingredients:

- 1 cup Greek yogurt
- 1/2 cup mixed berries (blueberries, strawberries)
- 2 tablespoons chopped nuts (almonds or walnuts)
- 1 tablespoon honey

Instructions:

1. In a glass, layer Greek yogurt, mixed berries, and chopped nuts.

2. Repeat the layers until the glass is filled.

3. Drizzle honey on top and savor the parfait.

Nutrition Information (per serving):

- Calories: 280

- Protein: 18g

- Carbohydrates: 25g

- Fat: 12g

- Fiber: 4g

- Sugar: 15g

- Portion Size: 1 serving

Sweet Potato and Black Bean Breakfast Burrito

Ingredients:

- 1 whole wheat tortilla

- 1/2 cup sweet potato, diced and roasted

- 1/4 cup black beans, cooked

- 2 large eggs, scrambled
- Salsa and avocado for topping

Instructions:

1. Fill the whole wheat tortilla with roasted sweet potato, black beans, and scrambled eggs.
2. Top with salsa and avocado.
3. Roll into a burrito and enjoy a satisfying breakfast.

Nutrition Information (per serving):

- Calories: 320
- Protein: 15g
- Carbohydrates: 40g
- Fat: 12g
- Fiber: 8g
- Sugar: 2g
- Portion Size: 1 serving

Whole Wheat Pancakes with Sugar-Free Syrup

Ingredients:

- 1 cup whole wheat flour
- 1 tablespoon baking powder
- 1/2 teaspoon cinnamon
- 1 cup almond milk
- 1 tablespoon apple cider vinegar
- Sugar-free syrup for serving

Instructions:

1. In a bowl, whisk together whole wheat flour, baking powder, and cinnamon.
2. In a separate bowl, mix almond milk and apple cider vinegar. Let it sit for a few minutes to create a "buttermilk."
3. Combine the wet and dry ingredients to form a batter.
4. Cook pancakes on a griddle until golden brown.
5. Serve with sugar-free syrup.

Nutrition Information (per serving):

- Calories: 250

- Protein: 8g

- Carbohydrates: 45g

- Fat: 4g

- Fiber: 6g

- Sugar: 2g

- Portion Size: 1 serving

Berry and Almond Smoothie Bowl

Ingredients:

- 1 cup mixed berries (strawberries, blueberries, raspberries)

- 1/2 banana, frozen

- 1/2 cup almond milk

- 2 tablespoons almond butter

- Toppings: sliced almonds, chia seeds, and fresh berries

Instructions:

1. Blend mixed berries, frozen banana, almond milk, and almond butter until smooth.

2. Pour into a bowl and add toppings of sliced almonds, chia seeds, and fresh berries.

Nutrition Information (per serving):

- Calories: 280
- Protein: 8g
- Carbohydrates: 30g
- Fat: 16g
- Fiber: 8g
- Sugar: 15g
- Portion Size: 1 serving

Overnight Oats with Cinnamon and Apples

Ingredients:

- 1/2 cup rolled oats
- 1/2 cup almond milk
- 1/2 apple, diced
- 1/2 teaspoon cinnamon
- 1 tablespoon maple syrup

Instructions:

1. In a jar, combine rolled oats, almond milk, diced apple, cinnamon, and maple syrup.

2. Stir well, cover, and refrigerate overnight.

3. In the morning, give it a good stir and enjoy the delicious and convenient overnight oats.

Nutrition Information (per serving):

- Calories: 220
- Protein: 6g
- Carbohydrates: 40g
- Fat: 4g
- Fiber: 8g
- Sugar: 15g
- Portion Size: 1 serving

Vegetable and Cheese Breakfast Quesadilla

Ingredients:

- 1 whole wheat tortilla
- 1/2 cup mixed bell peppers, diced
- 1/4 cup red onion, sliced
- 1/4 cup shredded cheese (cheddar or your choice)
- 1 teaspoon olive oil

Instructions:

1. In a pan, sauté bell peppers and red onion in olive oil until tender.
2. Place the whole wheat tortilla in the pan, add sautéed vegetables, and sprinkle with shredded cheese.
3. Fold the tortilla in half and cook until the cheese is melted.
4. Slice and enjoy a flavorful breakfast quesadilla.

Nutrition Information (per serving):

- Calories: 280
- Protein: 10g
- Carbohydrates: 30g
- Fat: 15g
- Fiber: 5g
- Sugar: 3g
- Portion Size: 1 serving

Pumpkin and Walnut Muffins

Ingredients:

- 1 cup whole wheat flour
- 1/2 cup canned pumpkin

- 1/4 cup chopped walnuts

- 1/4 cup maple syrup

- 1 teaspoon baking powder

- 1/2 teaspoon cinnamon

- 1/4 teaspoon nutmeg

- 1/4 teaspoon salt

- 1/4 cup unsweetened almond milk

- 1/4 cup coconut oil, melted

- 1 large egg

Instructions:

1. Preheat the oven to 350°F (175°C) and line a muffin tin with paper liners.

2. In a bowl, combine whole wheat flour, baking powder, cinnamon, nutmeg, and salt.

3. In another bowl, whisk together pumpkin, maple syrup, almond milk, coconut oil, and egg.

4. Add the wet ingredients to the dry ingredients and stir until just combined.

5. Fold in chopped walnuts.

6. Spoon the batter into the muffin tin and bake for 18-20 minutes or until a toothpick comes out clean.

7. Allow the muffins to cool before serving.

Nutrition Information (per serving):

- Calories: 180

- Protein: 4g

- Carbohydrates: 20g

- Fat: 10g

- Fiber: 3g

- Sugar: 6g

- Portion Size: 1 muffin

Blueberry Almond Baked Oatmeal

Ingredients:

- 1 cup rolled oats

- 1/2 cup almond milk

- 1/4 cup maple syrup

- 1/4 cup almond butter

- 1 teaspoon vanilla extract

- 1/2 teaspoon baking powder

- 1/4 teaspoon salt

- 1/2 cup blueberries (fresh or frozen)

- 1/4 cup sliced almonds

Instructions:

1. Preheat the oven to 350°F (175°C) and grease a baking dish.
2. In a bowl, mix rolled oats, almond milk, maple syrup, almond butter, vanilla extract, baking powder, and salt.
3. Fold in blueberries and spread the mixture in the baking dish.
4. Top with sliced almonds.
5. Bake for 25-30 minutes or until the edges are golden brown.
6. Allow it to cool slightly before serving.

Nutrition Information (per serving):

- Calories: 250
- Protein: 7g
- Carbohydrates: 30g
- Fat: 12g
- Fiber: 5g
- Sugar: 10g
- Portion Size: 1 serving

Broccoli and Cheese Mini Frittatas

Ingredients:

- 4 large eggs
- 1/2 cup broccoli florets, steamed and chopped
- 1/4 cup shredded cheddar cheese
- 1/4 cup milk (dairy or plant-based)
- Salt and pepper to taste
- Cooking spray

Instructions:

1. Preheat the oven to 375°F (190°C) and grease a muffin tin with cooking spray.
2. In a bowl, whisk together eggs, milk, salt, and pepper.
3. Stir in steamed and chopped broccoli and shredded cheddar cheese.
4. Pour the mixture into the muffin tin.
5. Bake for 15-20 minutes or until the frittatas are set.
6. Allow them to cool slightly before serving.

Nutrition Information (per serving):

- Calories: 180

- Protein: 12g

- Carbohydrates: 4g

- Fat: 12g

- Fiber: 1g

- Sugar: 1g

- Portion Size: 2 mini frittatas

Almond Butter and Banana Sandwich

Ingredients:

- 2 slices whole grain bread

- 2 tablespoons almond butter

- 1 banana, sliced

- 1 teaspoon honey (optional)

Instructions:

1. Spread almond butter evenly on one side of each slice of bread.

2. Place banana slices on one slice and drizzle with honey if desired.

3. Top with the other slice of bread to make a sandwich.

4. Slice in half and savor the delicious combination of almond butter and banana.

Nutrition Information (per serving):

- Calories: 350
- Protein: 8g
- Carbohydrates: 45g
- Fat: 16g
- Fiber: 8g
- Sugar: 15g
- Portion Size: 1 serving

Chapter 3: Lunch Recipes

These recipes are tailored for individuals with type 2 diabetes who follow a vegetarian lifestyle. Each dish is carefully crafted to balance taste and health, ensuring a satisfying dining experience while supporting your dietary needs.

Lentil and Vegetable Soup

Ingredients:

- 1 cup dry green or brown lentils
- 2 carrots, diced
- 1 zucchini, chopped
- 1 onion, finely chopped
- 3 cloves garlic, minced
- 1 can (14 oz) diced tomatoes
- 4 cups vegetable broth
- 1 teaspoon cumin
- Salt and pepper to taste

Instructions:

1. Rinse lentils thoroughly and set aside.

2. In a large pot, sauté onions and garlic until fragrant.

3. Add lentils, carrots, zucchini, diced tomatoes, vegetable broth, cumin, salt, and pepper.

4. Bring to a boil, then reduce heat and simmer until lentils are tender.

5. Serve hot and enjoy!

Nutrition Information:

- Calories: 250
- Protein: 15g
- Carbohydrates: 45g
- Fat: 2g
- Fiber: 18g
- Sugar: 6g
- Portion Size: 1 cup

Quinoa Salad with Roasted Vegetables

Ingredients:

- 1 cup quinoa, cooked
- 1 red bell pepper, sliced
- 1 yellow bell pepper, sliced
- 1 zucchini, sliced
- 1 cup cherry tomatoes, halved
- 2 tablespoons olive oil
- 1 teaspoon dried oregano
- Salt and pepper to taste

Instructions:

1. Preheat oven to 400°F (200°C).
2. Toss sliced vegetables with olive oil, oregano, salt, and pepper.
3. Roast in the oven until vegetables are tender.
4. Mix roasted vegetables with cooked quinoa.
5. Serve chilled or at room temperature.

Nutrition Information:

- Calories: 280

- Protein: 8g
- Carbohydrates: 45g
- Fat: 8g
- Fiber: 9g
- Sugar: 5g
- Portion Size: 1 cup

Chickpea and Spinach Stuffed Bell Peppers

Ingredients:

- 4 bell peppers, halved
- 1 can (15 oz) chickpeas, drained and rinsed
- 2 cups fresh spinach, chopped
- 1 cup cooked quinoa
- 1 onion, finely chopped
- 2 cloves garlic, minced
- 1 teaspoon cumin
- Salt and pepper to taste

Instructions:

1. Preheat oven to 375°F (190°C).

2. In a pan, sauté onions and garlic until translucent.

3. Add chickpeas, spinach, cooked quinoa, cumin, salt, and pepper.

4. Stuff bell peppers with the mixture and bake until peppers are tender.

5. Serve warm.

Nutrition Information:

- Calories: 220
- Protein: 10g
- Carbohydrates: 40g
- Fat: 4g
- Fiber: 10g
- Sugar: 8g
- Portion Size: 2 halves

Zucchini Noodles with Pesto and Cherry Tomatoes

Ingredients:

- 4 medium zucchinis, spiralized
- 1 cup cherry tomatoes, halved

- 1/2 cup fresh basil leaves

- 1/4 cup pine nuts

- 2 cloves garlic

- 1/3 cup grated Parmesan cheese (optional)

- 1/3 cup olive oil

- Salt and pepper to taste

Instructions:

1. Spiralize zucchinis to create noodles.

2. In a blender, combine basil, pine nuts, garlic, and Parmesan (if using).

3. Gradually add olive oil until a smooth pesto sauce forms.

4. Toss zucchini noodles with pesto and cherry tomatoes.

5. Season with salt and pepper, then serve.

Nutrition Information:

- Calories: 280

- Protein: 5g

- Carbohydrates: 10g

- Fat: 25g

- Fiber: 3g

- Sugar: 5g

- Portion Size: 1 cup

Brown Rice and Black Bean Burrito Bowl

Ingredients:

- 1 cup brown rice, cooked

- 1 can (15 oz) black beans, drained and rinsed

- 1 cup corn kernels

- 1 cup cherry tomatoes, quartered

- 1 avocado, diced

- 1/4 cup cilantro, chopped

- 1 lime, juiced

- Salt and pepper to taste

Instructions:

1. In a bowl, combine cooked brown rice, black beans, corn, cherry tomatoes, and avocado.

2. Add cilantro and lime juice, then toss.

3. Season with salt and pepper.

4. Serve at room temperature or chilled.

Nutrition Information:

- Calories: 320
- Protein: 10g
- Carbohydrates: 55g
- Fat: 8g
- Fiber: 12g
- Sugar: 3g
- Portion Size: 1 cup

Caprese Salad with Balsamic Glaze

Ingredients:

- 2 large tomatoes, sliced
- 1 ball fresh mozzarella, sliced
- 1/4 cup fresh basil leaves
- 2 tablespoons balsamic glaze
- Salt and pepper to taste

Instructions:

1. Arrange tomato and mozzarella slices on a platter.
2. Tuck fresh basil leaves between slices.

3. Drizzle with balsamic glaze and season with salt and pepper.

4. Serve as a refreshing Caprese salad.

Nutrition Information:

- Calories: 200
- Protein: 10g
- Carbohydrates: 5g
- Fat: 15g
- Fiber: 2g
- Sugar: 3g
- Portion Size: 1 cup

Grilled Eggplant and Hummus Wrap

Ingredients:

- 1 medium eggplant, sliced
- 4 whole-grain wraps
- 1 cup hummus
- 1 red onion, thinly sliced
- 2 cups arugula
- 2 tablespoons olive oil
- Salt and pepper to taste

Instructions:

1. Brush eggplant slices with olive oil and season with salt and pepper.
2. Grill the eggplant until tender and slightly charred.
3. Spread hummus on each wrap.
4. Layer grilled eggplant, red onion, and arugula.
5. Roll up the wraps and slice in half.

Nutrition Information:

- Calories: 320
- Protein: 10g
- Carbohydrates: 40g
- Fat: 15g
- Fiber: 8g
- Sugar: 5g
- Portion Size: 1 wrap

Cauliflower and Broccoli Quiche

Ingredients:

- 1 store-bought whole-grain pie crust
- 1 cup cauliflower florets, steamed
- 1 cup broccoli florets, steamed

- 1 cup shredded sharp cheddar cheese

- 4 large eggs

- 1 cup milk (or plant-based milk)

- Salt and pepper to taste

Instructions:

1. Preheat oven to 375°F (190°C).

2. Place pie crust in a pie dish.

3. Layer steamed cauliflower and broccoli in the crust.

4. Sprinkle shredded cheese over the vegetables.

5. In a bowl, whisk together eggs, milk, salt, and pepper.

6. Pour the egg mixture over the vegetables and cheese.

7. Bake for 30-35 minutes or until the center is set.

8. Allow to cool slightly before slicing.

Nutrition Information:

- Calories: 280

- Protein: 15g

- Carbohydrates: 20g

- Fat: 15g

- Fiber: 4g

- Sugar: 2g

- Portion Size: 1 slice

Cucumber and Avocado Sushi Rolls

Ingredients:

- 2 cups sushi rice, cooked

- 4 nori seaweed sheets

- 1 cucumber, julienned

- 1 avocado, sliced

- Soy sauce and wasabi for serving

Instructions:

1. Place a nori sheet on a bamboo sushi rolling mat.

2. Spread a thin layer of sushi rice over the nori, leaving a small border.

3. Arrange cucumber and avocado along the center of the rice.

4. Roll the sushi tightly using the bamboo mat.

5. Slice into bite-sized pieces.

6. Serve with soy sauce and wasabi.

Nutrition Information:

- Calories: 250
- Protein: 5g
- Carbohydrates: 50g
- Fat: 5g
- Fiber: 6g
- Sugar: 2g
- Portion Size: 6 pieces

Sweet Potato and Chickpea Curry

Ingredients:

- 2 sweet potatoes, peeled and diced
- 1 can (15 oz) chickpeas, drained and rinsed
- 1 onion, finely chopped
- 2 cloves garlic, minced
- 1 can (14 oz) diced tomatoes
- 1 can (14 oz) coconut milk
- 2 tablespoons curry powder
- Salt and pepper to taste

Instructions:

1. In a large pot, sauté onions and garlic until softened.

2. Add sweet potatoes, chickpeas, diced tomatoes, coconut milk, curry powder, salt, and pepper.

3. Simmer until sweet potatoes are tender.

4. Adjust seasoning as needed and serve hot.

Nutrition Information:

- Calories: 300
- Protein: 8g
- Carbohydrates: 45g
- Fat: 12g
- Fiber: 10g
- Sugar: 8g
- Portion Size: 1 cup

Mediterranean Chickpea Salad

Ingredients:

- 2 cans (15 oz each) chickpeas, drained and rinsed
- 1 cucumber, diced
- 1 cup cherry tomatoes, halved
- 1/2 cup Kalamata olives, sliced
- 1/2 cup crumbled feta cheese
- 1/4 cup red onion, finely chopped

- 2 tablespoons olive oil

- 1 teaspoon dried oregano

- Salt and pepper to taste

Instructions:

1. In a large bowl, combine chickpeas, cucumber, cherry tomatoes, olives, feta, and red onion.

2. Drizzle with olive oil and sprinkle with oregano, salt, and pepper.

3. Toss gently to combine.

4. Refrigerate for at least 30 minutes before serving.

Nutrition Information:

- Calories: 280

- Protein: 10g

- Carbohydrates: 30g

- Fat: 14g

- Fiber: 8g

- Sugar: 5g

- Portion Size: 1 cup

Spinach and Mushroom Quesadilla

Ingredients:

- 4 whole-grain tortillas
- 2 cups fresh spinach
- 1 cup mushrooms, sliced
- 1 cup shredded Monterey Jack cheese
- 1/2 cup salsa
- 1 tablespoon olive oil

Instructions:

1. In a pan, sauté mushrooms and spinach with olive oil until wilted.
2. Place a tortilla in a heated skillet.
3. Sprinkle with cheese and add a portion of the spinach and mushrooms.
4. Top with another tortilla and cook until the cheese is melted.
5. Repeat for the remaining tortillas.
6. Slice into wedges and serve with salsa.

Nutrition Information:

- Calories: 320

- Protein: 15g

- Carbohydrates: 30g

- Fat: 15g

- Fiber: 6g

- Sugar: 3g

- Portion Size: 1 quesadilla

Tomato Basil Bruschetta

Ingredients:

- 4 large tomatoes, diced

- 1/4 cup fresh basil, chopped

- 2 cloves garlic, minced

- 2 tablespoons balsamic vinegar

- 2 tablespoons olive oil

- Salt and pepper to taste

- Whole-grain baguette slices for serving

Instructions:

1. In a bowl, combine tomatoes, basil, garlic, balsamic vinegar, and olive oil.

2. Season with salt and pepper, then mix well.

3. Allow the mixture to marinate for at least 15 minutes.

4. Serve the tomato basil mixture on whole-grain baguette slices.

Nutrition Information:

- Calories: 180
- Protein: 3g
- Carbohydrates: 25g
- Fat: 8g
- Fiber: 5g
- Sugar: 8g
- Portion Size: 1/2 cup topping

Roasted Vegetable and Quinoa Stuffed Portobello Mushrooms

Ingredients:

- 4 large portobello mushrooms, cleaned and stems removed
- 1 cup quinoa, cooked
- 1 red bell pepper, diced
- 1 zucchini, diced
- 1 cup cherry tomatoes, halved

- 1/4 cup feta cheese, crumbled
- 2 tablespoons balsamic glaze
- 2 tablespoons olive oil
- Salt and pepper to taste

Instructions:

1. Preheat oven to 400°F (200°C).
2. Brush portobello mushrooms with olive oil and season with salt and pepper.
3. In a bowl, mix cooked quinoa, diced bell pepper, zucchini, cherry tomatoes, and feta.
4. Stuff the mushrooms with the quinoa mixture.
5. Roast in the oven until mushrooms are tender.
6. Drizzle with balsamic glaze before serving.

Nutrition Information:

- Calories: 250
- Protein: 10g
- Carbohydrates: 35g
- Fat: 10g
- Fiber: 6g
- Sugar: 5g

- Portion Size: 1 stuffed mushroom

Black Bean and Corn Quesadilla

Ingredients:

- 4 whole-grain tortillas
- 1 can (15 oz) black beans, drained and rinsed
- 1 cup corn kernels
- 1 cup shredded cheddar cheese
- 1/2 cup salsa
- 1 tablespoon olive oil

Instructions:

1. In a skillet, sauté black beans and corn with olive oil until heated through.
2. Place a tortilla in a heated skillet.
3. Sprinkle with cheese and add a portion of the black bean and corn mixture.
4. Top with another tortilla and cook until the cheese is melted.
5. Repeat for the remaining tortillas.
6. Slice into wedges and serve with salsa.

Nutrition Information:

- Calories: 310
- Protein: 15g
- Carbohydrates: 40g
- Fat: 12g
- Fiber: 8g
- Sugar: 3g
- Portion Size: 1 quesadilla

Chapter 4: Dinner Recipes

In this Chapter, where we delve into a delectable array of dinner recipes designed for those seeking a balance of flavor, nutrition, and diabetes-friendly goodness. These vegetarian delights are not only satisfying but also tailored to keep your blood sugar levels in check.

Baked Eggplant Parmesan

Ingredients:

- 1 large eggplant, sliced
- 1 cup whole wheat breadcrumbs
- 1 cup grated Parmesan cheese
- 2 cups marinara sauce
- 1 cup part-skim mozzarella cheese, shredded
- Fresh basil leaves for garnish

Instructions:

1. Preheat the oven to 375°F (190°C).
2. Dip eggplant slices in breadcrumbs and arrange in a single layer in a baking dish.

3. Bake until golden brown (about 20 minutes).

4. Layer eggplant with marinara, Parmesan, and mozzarella.

5. Repeat the layers and bake until bubbly and golden.

6. Garnish with fresh basil.

Nutrition Information (per serving):

- Calories: 280
- Protein: 15g
- Carbohydrates: 30g
- Fat: 12g
- Fiber: 8g
- Sugar: 12g
- Portion Size: 1 serving

Cauliflower Fried Rice with Tofu

Ingredients:

- 1 medium cauliflower, riced
- 1 cup tofu, cubed
- 1 cup mixed vegetables (peas, carrots, corn)
- 2 cloves garlic, minced
- 2 tbsp low-sodium soy sauce

- 1 tbsp sesame oil

- Green onions for garnish

Instructions:

1. Sauté tofu until golden.

2. Add garlic and mixed vegetables, stir-fry until tender.

3. Add cauliflower rice, soy sauce, and sesame oil.

4. Stir-fry until well combined.

5. Garnish with green onions.

Nutrition Information (per serving):

- Calories: 220

- Protein: 12g

- Carbohydrates: 18g

- Fat: 10g

- Fiber: 6g

- Sugar: 5g

- Portion Size: 1 serving

Stuffed Bell Peppers with Quinoa and Black Beans

Ingredients:

- 4 large bell peppers, halved
- 1 cup quinoa, cooked
- 1 can black beans, drained and rinsed
- 1 cup corn kernels
- 1 cup salsa
- 1 tsp cumin
- 1 cup shredded cheddar cheese

Instructions:

1. Preheat the oven to 375°F (190°C).
2. In a bowl, mix quinoa, black beans, corn, salsa, and cumin.
3. Stuff bell peppers with the quinoa mixture.
4. Top with shredded cheese.
5. Bake until peppers are tender (about 25 minutes).

Nutrition Information (per serving):

- Calories: 320
- Protein: 14g

- Carbohydrates: 45g

- Fat: 10g

- Fiber: 8g

- Sugar: 8g

- Portion Size: 1 serving

Spaghetti Squash Primavera

Ingredients:

- 1 medium spaghetti squash, halved

- 2 tbsp olive oil

- 2 cloves garlic, minced

- 1 cup cherry tomatoes, halved

- 1 cup broccoli florets

- 1 cup spinach leaves

- 1/4 cup grated Parmesan cheese

Instructions:

1. Preheat the oven to 400°F (200°C).

2. Roast spaghetti squash until fork-tender.

3. In a pan, sauté garlic, add tomatoes, broccoli, and spinach.

4. Scrape spaghetti squash into the pan, toss well.

5. Top with Parmesan and serve.

Nutrition Information (per serving):

- Calories: 180
- Protein: 5g
- Carbohydrates: 20g
- Fat: 10g
- Fiber: 6g
- Sugar: 5g
- Portion Size: 1 serving

Mushroom and Lentil Shepherd's Pie

Ingredients:

- 1 cup lentils, cooked
- 2 cups mushrooms, chopped
- 1 onion, diced
- 2 carrots, diced
- 2 cloves garlic, minced
- 1 cup vegetable broth
- 2 tbsp tomato paste
- Mashed sweet potatoes for topping

Instructions:

1. Sauté mushrooms, onion, and carrots until softened.

2. Add garlic, lentils, vegetable broth, and tomato paste.

3. Simmer until the mixture thickens.

4. Transfer to a baking dish, top with mashed sweet potatoes.

5. Bake until golden.

Nutrition Information (per serving):

- Calories: 250

- Protein: 12g

- Carbohydrates: 45g

- Fat: 4g

- Fiber: 10g

- Sugar: 8g

- Portion Size: 1 serving

Tofu and Vegetable Stir-Fry

Ingredients:

- 1 block tofu, cubed

- 2 cups broccoli florets

- 1 red bell pepper, sliced

- 1 carrot, julienned

- 2 tbsp soy sauce

- 1 tbsp hoisin sauce

- 1 tsp sesame oil

- Brown rice for serving

Instructions:

1. Sauté tofu until golden, set aside.

2. Stir-fry broccoli, bell pepper, and carrot.

3. Add tofu, soy sauce, hoisin sauce, and sesame oil.

4. Cook until well combined.

5. Serve over brown rice.

Nutrition Information (per serving):

- Calories: 280

- Protein: 18g

- Carbohydrates: 30g

- Fat: 12g

- Fiber: 8g

- Sugar: 5g

- Portion Size: 1 serving

Sweet Potato and Kale Gnocchi

Ingredients:

- 1 pound sweet potato gnocchi
- 2 cups kale, chopped
- 1/2 cup cherry tomatoes, halved
- 1/4 cup pine nuts, toasted
- 2 tbsp olive oil
- Salt and pepper to taste

Instructions:

1. Cook gnocchi according to package instructions.
2. In a pan, sauté kale and cherry tomatoes in olive oil.
3. Add cooked gnocchi and toss until heated through.
4. Season with salt and pepper.
5. Garnish with toasted pine nuts.

Nutrition Information (per serving):

- Calories: 320
- Protein: 8g
- Carbohydrates: 45g
- Fat: 14g
- Fiber: 6g

- Sugar: 5g

- Portion Size: 1 serving

Vegan Chili with Kidney Beans

Ingredients:

- 1 can kidney beans, drained and rinsed

- 1 can diced tomatoes

- 1 cup corn kernels

- 1 onion, diced

- 2 cloves garlic, minced

- 1 tbsp chili powder

- 1 tsp cumin

- Salt and pepper to taste

Instructions:

1. Sauté onion and garlic until fragrant.

2. Add kidney beans, diced tomatoes, corn, chili powder, and cumin.

3. Simmer until flavors meld.

4. Season with salt and pepper.

5. Serve hot.

Nutrition Information (per serving):

- Calories: 240
- Protein: 10g
- Carbohydrates: 40g
- Fat: 2g
- Fiber: 12g
- Sugar: 8g
- Portion Size: 1 serving

Portobello Mushroom Fajitas

Ingredients:

- 4 large portobello mushrooms, sliced
- 1 bell pepper, thinly sliced
- 1 onion, thinly sliced
- 2 tbsp fajita seasoning
- 2 tbsp olive oil
- Whole wheat tortillas for serving

Instructions:

1. Sauté mushrooms, bell pepper, and onion in olive oil.
2. Sprinkle fajita seasoning and toss until well-coated.
3. Cook until vegetables are tender.

4. Warm tortillas and fill with the mushroom mixture.

5. Serve with your favorite toppings.

Nutrition Information (per serving):

- Calories: 220

- Protein: 8g

- Carbohydrates: 30g

- Fat: 10g

- Fiber: 6g

- Sugar: 5g

- Portion Size: 1 serving

Lemon Garlic Asparagus and Quinoa

Ingredients:

- 1 cup quinoa, cooked

- 1 bunch asparagus, trimmed

- 2 cloves garlic, minced

- Zest and juice of 1 lemon

- 2 tbsp olive oil

- Salt and pepper to taste

Instructions:

1. Roast asparagus in olive oil until tender.

2. Sauté garlic until fragrant.

3. Toss cooked quinoa with asparagus, garlic, lemon zest, and juice.

4. Season with salt and pepper.

5. Serve as a light and refreshing dish.

Nutrition Information (per serving):

- Calories: 240

- Protein: 8g

- Carbohydrates: 35g

- Fat: 10g

- Fiber: 6g

- Sugar: 2g

- Portion Size: 1 serving

Ratatouille with Herbed Polenta

Ingredients:

- 1 eggplant, sliced

- 1 zucchini, sliced

- 1 yellow squash, sliced

- 1 bell pepper, diced

- 1 onion, sliced

- 2 cloves garlic, minced

- 2 cups tomato sauce

- 1 tsp dried herbs (thyme, rosemary, oregano)

- 1 cup polenta, cooked

- Fresh basil for garnish

Instructions:

1. Sauté onion and garlic until softened.
2. Layer sliced vegetables in a baking dish.
3. Pour tomato sauce over the vegetables.
4. Sprinkle with dried herbs.
5. Bake until vegetables are tender.
6. Serve over herbed polenta.
7. Garnish with fresh basil.

Nutrition Information (per serving):

- Calories: 280

- Protein: 8g

- Carbohydrates: 50g

- Fat: 6g

- Fiber: 10g

- Sugar: 12g

- Portion Size: 1 serving

Lentil and Vegetable Curry

Ingredients:

- 1 cup lentils, cooked

- 1 cup cauliflower florets

- 1 cup broccoli florets

- 1 carrot, sliced

- 1 onion, diced

- 2 cloves garlic, minced

- 1 can coconut milk

- 2 tbsp curry powder

- Fresh cilantro for garnish

Instructions:

1. Sauté onion and garlic until fragrant.

2. Add lentils, cauliflower, broccoli, carrot, coconut milk, and curry powder.

3. Simmer until vegetables are tender.

4. Garnish with fresh cilantro.

5. Serve over brown rice.

Nutrition Information (per serving):

- Calories: 320
- Protein: 14g
- Carbohydrates: 40g
- Fat: 10g
- Fiber: 12g
- Sugar: 8g
- Portion Size: 1 serving

Stuffed Acorn Squash with Wild Rice

Ingredients:

- 2 acorn squash, halved
- 1 cup wild rice, cooked
- 1 cup cranberries, dried
- 1/2 cup pecans, chopped
- 1/4 cup maple syrup
- 1 tsp cinnamon
- 1 tbsp olive oil

Instructions:

1. Roast acorn squash halves until tender.
2. In a bowl, mix wild rice, cranberries, pecans, maple syrup, and cinnamon.
3. Stuff each squash half with the rice mixture.
4. Drizzle with olive oil.
5. Bake until golden and fragrant.

Nutrition Information (per serving):

- Calories: 280
- Protein: 6g
- Carbohydrates: 50g
- Fat: 8g
- Fiber: 8g
- Sugar: 15g
- Portion Size: 1 serving

Brussels Sprouts and Pecan Salad

Ingredients:

- 2 cups Brussels sprouts, shaved
- 1/2 cup pecans, toasted
- 1/4 cup dried cranberries

- 1/4 cup feta cheese, crumbled

- 2 tbsp balsamic vinaigrette

- Salt and pepper to taste

Instructions:

1. In a bowl, combine shaved Brussels sprouts, toasted pecans, cranberries, and feta.

2. Drizzle with balsamic vinaigrette.

3. Toss until well-coated.

4. Season with salt and pepper.

5. Serve as a refreshing salad.

Nutrition Information (per serving):

- Calories: 220

- Protein: 6g

- Carbohydrates: 20g

- Fat: 15g

- Fiber: 6g

- Sugar: 8g

- Portion Size: 1 serving

Butternut Squash and Sage Risotto

Ingredients:

- 1 cup Arborio rice
- 2 cups butternut squash, diced
- 1 onion, finely chopped
- 2 cloves garlic, minced
- 4 cups vegetable broth, warm
- 1/2 cup white wine
- 2 tbsp fresh sage, chopped
- 2 tbsp olive oil

Instructions:

1. Sauté onion and garlic until translucent.
2. Add Arborio rice, stir until coated with oil.
3. Pour in white wine and cook until absorbed.
4. Gradually add warm vegetable broth, stirring continuously.
5. Stir in butternut squash and sage.
6. Cook until rice is creamy and squash is tender.
7. Drizzle with olive oil before serving.

Nutrition Information (per serving):

- Calories: 300
- Protein: 6g
- Carbohydrates: 55g
- Fat: 8g
- Fiber: 6g
- Sugar: 5g
- Portion Size: 1 serving

Chapter 5: Snacks and Appetizers

In this chapter, we present a collection of snacks and appetizers that not only satisfy your taste buds but also align with dietary guidelines for diabetes management.

Guacamole with Vegetable Sticks

Ingredients:

- 2 ripe avocados
- 1 small red onion, finely diced
- 1 medium tomato, diced
- 1 clove garlic, minced
- 1 lime, juiced
- Salt and pepper to taste
- Assorted vegetable sticks (carrots, bell peppers, cucumber)

Instructions:

1. In a bowl, mash the avocados with a fork.
2. Add diced red onion, tomato, minced garlic, lime juice, salt, and pepper. Mix well.

3. Serve the guacamole with colorful vegetable sticks.

Nutrition Information (per serving):

- Calories: 120
- Protein: 2g
- Carbohydrates: 8g
- Fat: 10g
- Fiber: 5g
- Sugar: 1g
- Portion size: 1/2 cup guacamole with vegetable sticks

Baked Sweet Potato Fries

Ingredients:

- 2 large sweet potatoes, cut into fries
- 1 tablespoon olive oil
- 1 teaspoon paprika
- 1 teaspoon garlic powder
- Salt and pepper to taste

Instructions:

1. Preheat the oven to 425°F (220°C).

2. In a bowl, toss sweet potato fries with olive oil, paprika, garlic powder, salt, and pepper.

3. Spread the fries on a baking sheet and bake for 25-30 minutes, turning once.

Nutrition Information (per serving):

- Calories: 150

- Protein: 2g

- Carbohydrates: 30g

- Fat: 3g

- Fiber: 5g

- Sugar: 6g

- Portion size: 1 cup baked sweet potato fries

Hummus and Whole Grain Crackers

Ingredients:

- 1 can (15 oz) chickpeas, drained

- 2 tablespoons tahini

- 2 tablespoons olive oil

- 1 clove garlic, minced

- 1 lemon, juiced

- Whole grain crackers

Instructions:

1. In a food processor, blend chickpeas, tahini, olive oil, minced garlic, and lemon juice until smooth.

2. Serve the hummus with whole grain crackers.

Nutrition Information (per serving):

- Calories: 160
- Protein: 5g
- Carbohydrates: 18g
- Fat: 8g
- Fiber: 5g
- Sugar: 1g
- Portion size: 1/4 cup hummus with whole grain crackers

Greek Yogurt and Berry Popsicles

Ingredients:

- 1 cup Greek yogurt
- 1 cup mixed berries (strawberries, blueberries, raspberries)
- 2 tablespoons honey

Instructions:

1. In a blender, mix Greek yogurt, mixed berries, and honey until well combined.

2. Pour the mixture into popsicle molds and freeze for at least 4 hours.

Nutrition Information (per serving):

- Calories: 90

- Protein: 6g

- Carbohydrates: 15g

- Fat: 1g

- Fiber: 2g

- Sugar: 11g

- Portion size: 1 popsicle

Edamame and Sea Salt

Ingredients:

- 2 cups edamame (shelled)

- Sea salt to taste

Instructions:

1. Steam or boil the edamame until tender.

2. Sprinkle with sea salt and toss to coat.

Nutrition Information (per serving):

- Calories: 150
- Protein: 13g
- Carbohydrates: 11g
- Fat: 7g
- Fiber: 8g
- Sugar: 3g
- Portion size: 1 cup edamame

Roasted Chickpeas with Paprika

Ingredients:

- 2 cans (15 oz each) chickpeas, drained and rinsed
- 2 tablespoons olive oil
- 1 teaspoon paprika
- 1/2 teaspoon cayenne pepper
- Salt to taste

Instructions:

1. Preheat the oven to 400°F (200°C).

2. Toss chickpeas with olive oil, paprika, cayenne pepper, and salt.

3. Spread on a baking sheet and roast for 25-30 minutes until crispy.

Nutrition Information (per serving):

- Calories: 180

- Protein: 7g

- Carbohydrates: 25g

- Fat: 6g

- Fiber: 7g

- Sugar: 4g

- Portion size: 1/2 cup roasted chickpeas

Avocado Salsa with Whole Grain Tortilla Chips

Ingredients:

- 2 avocados, diced

- 1 cup cherry tomatoes, halved

- 1/4 cup red onion, finely chopped

- 1/4 cup cilantro, chopped

- 1 lime, juiced

- Whole grain tortilla chips

Instructions:

1. In a bowl, combine diced avocados, cherry tomatoes, red onion, cilantro, and lime juice.

2. Serve with whole grain tortilla chips.

Nutrition Information (per serving):

- Calories: 160

- Protein: 3g

- Carbohydrates: 18g

- Fat: 10g

- Fiber: 6g

- Sugar: 2g

- Portion size: 1/2 cup avocado salsa with tortilla chips

Cucumber Rolls with Herbed Cream Cheese

Ingredients:

- 2 large cucumbers, thinly sliced lengthwise

- 1 cup cream cheese, softened

- 2 tablespoons fresh dill, chopped

- Salt and pepper to taste

Instructions:

1. In a bowl, mix softened cream cheese with chopped dill, salt, and pepper.

2. Spread a thin layer of herbed cream cheese on cucumber slices and roll them up.

Nutrition Information (per serving):

- Calories: 120

- Protein: 3g

- Carbohydrates: 5g

- Fat: 10g

- Fiber: 1g

- Sugar: 2g

- Portion size: 4 cucumber rolls

Nut Mix with Dried Fruits

Ingredients:

- 1 cup mixed nuts (almonds, walnuts, pistachios)

- 1/2 cup dried fruits (apricots, cranberries, raisins)

Instructions:

1. Combine mixed nuts and dried fruits in a bowl.
2. Toss to mix well.

Nutrition Information (per serving):

- Calories: 200
- Protein: 5g
- Carbohydrates: 18g
- Fat: 13g
- Fiber: 4g
- Sugar: 10g
- Portion size: 1/2 cup nut mix with dried fruits

Stuffed Mushrooms with Spinach and Feta

Ingredients:

- 12 large mushrooms, stems removed
- 2 cups spinach, chopped
- 1/2 cup feta cheese, crumbled

- 2 cloves garlic, minced
- 1 tablespoon olive oil

Instructions:

1. Preheat the oven to 375°F (190°C).
2. In a pan, sauté spinach and garlic in olive oil until wilted.
3. Stuff mushroom caps with the spinach mixture and top with crumbled feta.
4. Bake for 15-20 minutes until mushrooms are tender.

Nutrition Information (per serving):

- Calories: 90
- Protein: 5g
- Carbohydrates: 5g
- Fat: 6g
- Fiber: 2g
- Sugar: 2g
- Portion size: 3 stuffed mushrooms

Caprese Skewers with Balsamic Glaze

Ingredients:

- Cherry tomatoes
- Fresh mozzarella balls
- Fresh basil leaves
- Balsamic glaze

Instructions:

1. Thread cherry tomatoes, mozzarella balls, and basil leaves onto skewers.
2. Drizzle with balsamic glaze before serving.

Nutrition Information (per serving):

- Calories: 80
- Protein: 5g
- Carbohydrates: 3g
- Fat: 6g
- Fiber: 1g
- Sugar: 2g
- Portion size: 4 skewers

Beet and Goat Cheese Crostini

Ingredients:

- Baguette slices, toasted
- Roasted beets, sliced
- Goat cheese
- Honey for drizzling

Instructions:

1. Top toasted baguette slices with roasted beet slices and crumbled goat cheese.
2. Drizzle with honey before serving.

Nutrition Information (per serving):

- Calories: 120
- Protein: 4g
- Carbohydrates: 15g
- Fat: 5g
- Fiber: 2g
- Sugar: 5g
- Portion size: 3 crostini

Apple Slices with Almond Butter

Ingredients:

- 2 apples, sliced
- Almond butter for dipping

Instructions:

1. Arrange apple slices on a plate.
2. Serve with a side of almond butter for dipping.

Nutrition Information (per serving):

- Calories: 160
- Protein: 4g
- Carbohydrates: 25g
- Fat: 7g
- Fiber: 6g
- Sugar: 18g
- Portion size: 1 apple with almond butter

Kale Chips with Nutritional Yeast

Ingredients:

- 1 bunch kale, stems removed and torn into pieces

- 1 tablespoon olive oil

- 2 tablespoons nutritional yeast

- Salt to taste

Instructions:

1. Preheat the oven to 350°F (175°C).

2. Toss kale pieces with olive oil, nutritional yeast, and salt.

3. Bake for 10-15 minutes until crispy.

Nutrition Information (per serving):

- Calories: 70

- Protein: 3g

- Carbohydrates: 8g

- Fat: 4g

- Fiber: 3g

- Sugar: 1g

- Portion size: 1 cup kale chips

Mango and Black Bean Salsa

Ingredients:

- 1 ripe mango, diced

- 1 can (15 oz) black beans, drained and rinsed
- 1/2 red onion, finely chopped
- 1 jalapeño, seeded and minced
- Fresh cilantro, chopped
- Lime juice to taste

Instructions:

1. In a bowl, combine diced mango, black beans, red onion, jalapeño, cilantro, and lime juice.
2. Mix well and refrigerate for at least 30 minutes before serving.

Nutrition Information (per serving):

- Calories: 130
- Protein: 6g
- Carbohydrates: 25g
- Fat: 1g
- Fiber: 7g
- Sugar: 6g
- Portion size: 1/2 cup salsa

Chapter 6: Desserts

This chapter brings you a collection of scrumptious desserts designed with your well-being in mind. From the burst of berries to the richness of dark chocolate, each recipe is crafted to satisfy your sweet tooth while keeping a check on your nutritional needs.

Berry and Almond Crisp

Ingredients:

- 2 cups mixed berries (strawberries, blueberries, raspberries)
- 1/2 cup almond flour
- 1/4 cup rolled oats
- 2 tablespoons coconut oil
- 2 tablespoons maple syrup
- 1/4 teaspoon cinnamon
- Pinch of salt

Instructions:

1. Preheat oven to 350°F (175°C).

2. In a bowl, mix berries and place them in a baking dish.

3. In another bowl, combine almond flour, rolled oats, coconut oil, maple syrup, cinnamon, and salt.

4. Sprinkle the almond mixture over the berries.

5. Bake for 25-30 minutes or until the topping is golden brown.

6. Serve warm, and enjoy!

Nutrition Information (per serving):

- Calories: 180
- Protein: 3g
- Carbohydrates: 22g
- Fat: 10g
- Fiber: 5g
- Sugar: 10g
- Portion Size: 1 cup

Dark Chocolate Avocado Mousse

Ingredients:

- 2 ripe avocados
- 1/2 cup unsweetened cocoa powder

- 1/4 cup maple syrup

- 1/4 cup almond milk

- 1 teaspoon vanilla extract

- Pinch of salt

Instructions:

1. In a blender, combine avocados, cocoa powder, maple syrup, almond milk, vanilla extract, and salt.

2. Blend until smooth and creamy.

3. Refrigerate for at least 2 hours before serving.

4. Garnish with berries or nuts if desired.

5. Delight in the velvety goodness!

Nutrition Information (per serving):

- Calories: 220

- Protein: 4g

- Carbohydrates: 18g

- Fat: 15g

- Fiber: 8g

- Sugar: 6g

- Portion Size: 1/2 cup

Coconut Chia Seed Pudding

Ingredients:

- 1/4 cup chia seeds
- 1 cup coconut milk
- 1 tablespoon maple syrup
- 1/2 teaspoon vanilla extract
- Fresh berries for topping

Instructions:

1. In a bowl, mix chia seeds, coconut milk, maple syrup, and vanilla extract.
2. Stir well, cover, and refrigerate overnight.
3. Before serving, stir the pudding and top with fresh berries.
4. Enjoy the creamy goodness!

Nutrition Information (per serving):

- Calories: 180
- Protein: 4g
- Carbohydrates: 15g
- Fat: 12g
- Fiber: 8g

- Sugar: 5g

- Portion Size: 1/2 cup

Baked Apple with Cinnamon

Ingredients:

- 2 apples, cored and halved

- 1 tablespoon cinnamon

- 1 tablespoon coconut oil

- 2 tablespoons chopped nuts (walnuts or almonds)

Instructions:

1. Preheat oven to 375°F (190°C).

2. Place apple halves on a baking sheet.

3. Sprinkle with cinnamon and dot with coconut oil.

4. Bake for 20-25 minutes until apples are tender.

5. Garnish with chopped nuts and serve warm.

Nutrition Information (per serving):

- Calories: 120

- Protein: 1g

- Carbohydrates: 18g

- Fat: 6g

- Fiber: 4g

- Sugar: 12g

- Portion Size: 1 apple half

Vegan Chocolate Chip Cookies

Ingredients:

- 1 cup almond flour

- 1/4 cup coconut flour

- 1/4 cup coconut oil, melted

- 1/4 cup maple syrup

- 1/2 teaspoon baking soda

- 1/4 teaspoon salt

- 1/2 cup dairy-free chocolate chips

Instructions:

1. Preheat oven to 350°F (175°C).

2. In a bowl, combine almond flour, coconut flour, melted coconut oil, maple syrup, baking soda, and salt.

3. Fold in chocolate chips.

4. Drop spoonfuls onto a baking sheet and flatten each cookie.

5. Bake for 10-12 minutes or until edges are golden.

6. Allow to cool before serving.

Nutrition Information (per serving, 2 cookies):

- Calories: 180

- Protein: 3g

- Carbohydrates: 15g

- Fat: 12g

- Fiber: 2g

- Sugar: 8g

- Portion Size: 2 cookies

Almond Flour Banana Bread

Ingredients:

- 2 ripe bananas, mashed

- 3 eggs

- 1/4 cup coconut oil, melted

- 1 teaspoon vanilla extract

- 2 cups almond flour

- 1 teaspoon baking powder

- 1/2 teaspoon cinnamon

- Pinch of salt

Instructions:

1. Preheat oven to 350°F (175°C). Grease a loaf pan.

2. In a bowl, combine mashed bananas, eggs, melted coconut oil, and vanilla extract.

3. In another bowl, mix almond flour, baking powder, cinnamon, and salt.

4. Combine wet and dry ingredients, pour into the loaf pan, and smooth the top.

5. Bake for 45-50 minutes or until a toothpick comes out clean.

6. Allow to cool before slicing.

Nutrition Information (per serving, 1 slice):

- Calories: 180
- Protein: 5g
- Carbohydrates: 14g
- Fat: 12g
- Fiber: 3g
- Sugar: 6g
- Portion Size: 1 slice

Strawberry Shortcake with Almond Flour Biscuits

Ingredients:

- 2 cups sliced strawberries
- 1 tablespoon maple syrup
- 1 1/2 cups almond flour
- 1/4 cup coconut flour
- 1/4 cup coconut oil, solid
- 1/4 cup almond milk
- 1 teaspoon baking powder
- 1/2 teaspoon vanilla extract
- Pinch of salt

Instructions:

1. In a bowl, mix sliced strawberries with maple syrup and set aside.
2. Preheat oven to 350°F (175°C).
3. In a separate bowl, combine almond flour, coconut flour, solid coconut oil, almond milk, baking powder, vanilla extract, and salt.
4. Form biscuit shapes and place on a baking sheet.
5. Bake for 15-18 minutes or until golden.

6. Assemble shortcakes with sliced strawberries.

Nutrition Information (per serving, 1 shortcake):
- Calories: 200
- Protein: 4g
- Carbohydrates: 18g
- Fat: 14g
- Fiber: 4g
- Sugar: 6g
- Portion Size: 1 shortcake

Pistachio and Raspberry Energy Bites

Ingredients:
- 1 cup shelled pistachios
- 1 cup dried raspberries
- 1/4 cup almond butter
- 1/4 cup honey
- 1 teaspoon vanilla extract
- Pinch of salt
- Shredded coconut for coating

Instructions:

1. In a food processor, blend pistachios until finely ground.
2. Add dried raspberries, almond butter, honey, vanilla extract, and salt. Blend until a dough-like consistency forms.
3. Roll the mixture into bite-sized balls and coat with shredded coconut.
4. Refrigerate for at least 30 minutes before serving.

Nutrition Information (per serving, 2 energy bites):

- Calories: 160
- Protein: 4g
- Carbohydrates: 16g
- Fat: 9g
- Fiber: 3g
- Sugar: 10g
- Portion Size: 2 energy bites

Blueberry and Lemon Frozen Yogurt

Ingredients:

- 2 cups frozen blueberries

- 1 cup Greek yogurt
- 1/4 cup honey
- Zest of 1 lemon
- 1 tablespoon lemon juice

Instructions:

1. In a blender, combine frozen blueberries, Greek yogurt, honey, lemon zest, and lemon juice.
2. Blend until smooth.
3. Transfer the mixture to a container and freeze for at least 4 hours.
4. Scoop and enjoy this refreshing frozen treat.

Nutrition Information (per serving):

- Calories: 120
- Protein: 5g
- Carbohydrates: 20g
- Fat: 2g
- Fiber: 3g
- Sugar: 15g
- Portion Size: 1/2 cup

Pumpkin Pie Smoothie Bowl

Ingredients:

- 1 cup canned pumpkin puree
- 1 frozen banana
- 1/2 cup almond milk
- 1 tablespoon maple syrup
- 1/2 teaspoon pumpkin spice
- Granola and sliced almonds for topping

Instructions:

1. In a blender, combine pumpkin puree, frozen banana, almond milk, maple syrup, and pumpkin spice.
2. Blend until smooth and creamy.
3. Pour into a bowl and top with granola and sliced almonds.
4. Dive into the autumn flavors!

Nutrition Information (per serving):

- Calories: 200
- Protein: 5g
- Carbohydrates: 25g
- Fat: 8g

- Fiber: 6g

- Sugar: 12g

- Portion Size: 1 bowl

Avocado Lime Cheesecake

Ingredients:

- 2 ripe avocados

- 1 cup cashews, soaked

- 1/2 cup coconut cream

- 1/4 cup lime juice

- 1/4 cup maple syrup

- 1 teaspoon vanilla extract

- Zest of 1 lime

- 1/4 cup coconut oil, melted

- Almond crust (almond flour, melted coconut oil, and a pinch of salt)

Instructions:

1. Prepare the almond crust by combining almond flour, melted coconut oil, and a pinch of salt. Press into the base of a springform pan.

2. In a blender, blend avocados, soaked cashews, coconut cream, lime juice, maple syrup, vanilla extract, and lime zest until smooth.

3. Add melted coconut oil and blend again.

4. Pour the mixture over the almond crust.

5. Refrigerate for at least 4 hours or until set.

6. Slice and enjoy this creamy, lime-infused delight!

Nutrition Information (per serving, 1 slice):

- Calories: 250
- Protein: 5g
- Carbohydrates: 18g
- Fat: 20g
- Fiber: 5g
- Sugar: 8g
- Portion Size: 1 slice

Chocolate Covered Strawberries

Ingredients:

- 1 cup dark chocolate chips
- 1 tablespoon coconut oil
- 16 strawberries, washed and dried

Instructions:

1. In a microwave-safe bowl, melt dark chocolate chips and coconut oil in 30-second intervals, stirring between each interval.
2. Dip each strawberry into the melted chocolate, ensuring it's well-coated.
3. Place on a parchment-lined tray and refrigerate until the chocolate hardens.
4. Enjoy these decadent chocolate-covered strawberries guilt-free!

Nutrition Information (per serving, 4 strawberries):

- Calories: 150
- Protein: 2g
- Carbohydrates: 20g
- Fat: 9g
- Fiber: 4g
- Sugar: 12g
- Portion Size: 4 strawberries

Raspberry Almond Tart

Ingredients:

- 1 1/2 cups almond flour
- 1/4 cup coconut flour
- 1/4 cup coconut oil, melted
- 2 tablespoons maple syrup
- 1 cup fresh raspberries

Instructions:

1. Preheat oven to 350°F (175°C).
2. In a bowl, combine almond flour, coconut flour, melted coconut oil, and maple syrup.
3. Press the mixture into a tart pan to form the crust.
4. Bake for 10-12 minutes or until golden brown.
5. Allow the crust to cool, then fill with fresh raspberries.
6. Refrigerate for at least 2 hours before serving.

Nutrition Information (per serving, 1 slice):

- Calories: 180
- Protein: 4g
- Carbohydrates: 15g

- Fat: 12g
- Fiber: 5g
- Sugar: 6g
- Portion Size: 1 slice

Mango Sorbet with Mint

Ingredients:

- 2 cups frozen mango chunks
- 1/4 cup fresh mint leaves
- 1/4 cup coconut water
- 1 tablespoon lime juice
- 2 tablespoons agave nectar

Instructions:

1. In a blender, blend frozen mango chunks, mint leaves, coconut water, lime juice, and agave nectar until smooth.
2. Transfer the mixture to a container and freeze for at least 4 hours.
3. Scoop and enjoy this refreshing mango sorbet.

Nutrition Information (per serving):

- Calories: 120
- Protein: 1g
- Carbohydrates: 30g
- Fat: 0g
- Fiber: 3g
- Sugar: 25g
- Portion Size: 1/2 cup

Vanilla Bean Coconut Rice Pudding

Ingredients:

- 1 cup cooked brown rice
- 1 can (14 oz) coconut milk
- 1/4 cup maple syrup
- 1 vanilla bean, seeds scraped
- 1/4 teaspoon cinnamon
- Pinch of salt

Instructions:

1. In a saucepan, combine cooked brown rice, coconut milk, maple syrup, vanilla bean seeds, cinnamon, and a pinch of salt.

2. Cook over medium heat, stirring frequently, until the mixture thickens.

3. Remove from heat and let it cool.

4. Serve chilled and savor the delightful flavors!

Nutrition Information (per serving, 1/2 cup):

- Calories: 180
- Protein: 2g
- Carbohydrates: 20g
- Fat: 10g
- Fiber: 1g
- Sugar: 10g
- Portion Size: 1/2 cup

Chapter 7: Smoothies

These smoothies are crafted with a thoughtful blend of ingredients, ensuring a delightful fusion of flavors and a burst of nutrition in every sip.

Green Goddess Smoothie with Spinach and Kale

Ingredients:

- 1 cup fresh spinach leaves
- 1/2 cup kale, chopped
- 1 green apple, cored and chopped
- 1/2 cucumber, peeled and sliced
- 1/2 lemon, juiced
- 1 cup coconut water
- Ice cubes (optional)

Instructions:

1. In a blender, combine spinach, kale, apple, cucumber, and lemon juice.
2. Add coconut water and blend until smooth.

3. If desired, add ice cubes and blend again.

4. Pour into a glass and enjoy!

Nutrition Information (per serving):

- Calories: 90
- Protein: 3g
- Carbohydrates: 20g
- Fat: 1g
- Fiber: 5g
- Sugar: 10g
- Portion Size: 1 serving

Berry Blast Smoothie with Chia Seeds

Ingredients:

- 1 cup mixed berries (strawberries, blueberries, raspberries)
- 1 banana, frozen
- 1 tablespoon chia seeds
- 1/2 cup Greek yogurt
- 1 cup almond milk

- Honey to taste

Instructions:

1. Combine mixed berries, frozen banana, chia seeds, Greek yogurt, and almond milk in a blender.
2. Blend until smooth.
3. Add honey to taste and blend again.
4. Pour into a glass and savor the berry goodness!

Nutrition Information (per serving):

- Calories: 150
- Protein: 7g
- Carbohydrates: 25g
- Fat: 4g
- Fiber: 6g
- Sugar: 15g
- Portion Size: 1 serving

Tropical Paradise Smoothie with Pineapple and Coconut

Ingredients:

- 1 cup pineapple chunks
- 1/2 cup mango, diced
- 1/4 cup shredded coconut
- 1/2 cup vanilla Greek yogurt
- 1 cup coconut water
- Ice cubes (optional)

Instructions:

1. Blend pineapple, mango, shredded coconut, Greek yogurt, and coconut water until smooth.
2. Add ice cubes if desired and blend again.
3. Pour into a tropical glass and transport yourself to paradise!

Nutrition Information (per serving):

- Calories: 120
- Protein: 5g
- Carbohydrates: 25g
- Fat: 2g

- Fiber: 4g

- Sugar: 18g

- Portion Size: 1 serving

Almond Butter Banana Smoothie

Ingredients:

- 2 ripe bananas

- 2 tablespoons almond butter

- 1 cup almond milk

- 1/2 teaspoon vanilla extract

- Ice cubes (optional)

Instructions:

1. Peel and slice the bananas.

2. In a blender, combine bananas, almond butter, almond milk, and vanilla extract.

3. Blend until creamy and smooth.

4. Add ice cubes if you prefer a chilled texture.

5. Pour into a glass and relish the delightful almond and banana fusion!

Nutrition Information (per serving):

- Calories: 220
- Protein: 5g
- Carbohydrates: 30g
- Fat: 11g
- Fiber: 5g
- Sugar: 14g
- Portion Size: 1 serving

Mango Tango Smoothie with Turmeric

Ingredients:

- 1 cup fresh mango chunks
- 1/2 banana
- 1/2 teaspoon turmeric powder
- 1/2 cup plain yogurt
- 1/2 cup orange juice
- Dash of black pepper (optional)

Instructions:

1. Blend mango chunks, banana, turmeric powder, yogurt, and orange juice until smooth.
2. Add a dash of black pepper if you desire a subtle kick.
3. Pour into a glass and dance with the mango tango!

Nutrition Information (per serving):

- Calories: 160
- Protein: 4g
- Carbohydrates: 35g
- Fat: 1g
- Fiber: 3g
- Sugar: 25g
- Portion Size: 1 serving

Blueberry and Oatmeal Power Smoothie

Ingredients:

- 1/2 cup blueberries (fresh or frozen)
- 1/4 cup rolled oats

- 1/2 cup Greek yogurt

- 1 tablespoon honey

- 1 cup almond milk

Instructions:

1. Blend blueberries, rolled oats, Greek yogurt, honey, and almond milk until well combined.

2. Pour into a glass and enjoy the nourishing power of blueberries and oats!

Nutrition Information (per serving):

- Calories: 180

- Protein: 8g

- Carbohydrates: 30g

- Fat: 4g

- Fiber: 5g

- Sugar: 15g

- Portion Size: 1 serving

Spinach and Pineapple Detox Smoothie

Ingredients:

- 1 cup fresh spinach leaves
- 1/2 cup pineapple chunks
- 1/2 cucumber, peeled and sliced
- 1/2 lemon, juiced
- 1 tablespoon fresh ginger, grated
- 1 cup coconut water
- Ice cubes (optional)

Instructions:

1. Blend spinach, pineapple, cucumber, lemon juice, ginger, and coconut water until smooth.
2. Add ice cubes if desired and blend again.
3. Pour into a glass and refresh with this detoxifying green elixir!

Nutrition Information (per serving):

- Calories: 70
- Protein: 2g
- Carbohydrates: 18g

- Fat: 1g

- Fiber: 4g

- Sugar: 10g

- Portion Size: 1 serving

Peach and Ginger Smoothie

Ingredients:

- 1 cup sliced peaches (fresh or frozen)

- 1/2 inch fresh ginger, peeled and grated

- 1/2 cup vanilla Greek yogurt

- 1/2 cup almond milk

- 1 tablespoon honey

- Ice cubes (optional)

Instructions:

1. Blend sliced peaches, grated ginger, Greek yogurt, almond milk, and honey until smooth.

2. Add ice cubes if you prefer a chilled texture.

3. Pour into a glass and savor the delightful peach and ginger combination!

Nutrition Information (per serving):

- Calories: 130
- Protein: 5g
- Carbohydrates: 25g
- Fat: 3g
- Fiber: 3g
- Sugar: 20g
- Portion Size: 1 serving

Cucumber Mint Cooler Smoothie

Ingredients:

- 1/2 cucumber, peeled and sliced
- 1/4 cup fresh mint leaves
- 1/2 lime, juiced
- 1 tablespoon honey
- 1 cup coconut water
- Ice cubes (optional)

Instructions:

1. Blend cucumber, mint leaves, lime juice, honey, and coconut water until well combined.
2. Add ice cubes if desired and blend again.

3. Pour into a glass and enjoy the cool and refreshing
   sensation!

Nutrition Information (per serving):

- Calories: 60
- Protein: 1g
- Carbohydrates: 15g
- Fat: 0g
- Fiber: 2g
- Sugar: 10g
- Portion Size: 1 serving

Chocolate Avocado Protein Smoothie

Ingredients:

- 1/2 avocado, peeled and pitted
- 1 scoop chocolate protein powder
- 1 tablespoon unsweetened cocoa powder
- 1 cup almond milk
- 1 tablespoon chia seeds
- Ice cubes (optional)

Instructions:

1. Blend avocado, chocolate protein powder, cocoa powder, almond milk, and chia seeds until smooth.
2. Add ice cubes if you desire a colder texture.
3. Pour into a glass and indulge in this creamy chocolate delight packed with protein!

Nutrition Information (per serving):

- Calories: 250
- Protein: 20g
- Carbohydrates: 18g
- Fat: 15g
- Fiber: 8g
- Sugar: 3g
- Portion Size: 1 serving

Golden Turmeric Latte Smoothie

Ingredients:

- 1 banana, frozen
- 1/2 teaspoon turmeric powder
- 1/2 teaspoon cinnamon
- 1/2 teaspoon ginger, grated

- 1 cup coconut milk

- 1 teaspoon honey

Instructions:

1. Blend frozen banana, turmeric powder, cinnamon, grated ginger, coconut milk, and honey until smooth.

2. Pour into a glass and enjoy the golden goodness of this turmeric latte smoothie!

Nutrition Information (per serving):

- Calories: 180

- Protein: 2g

- Carbohydrates: 30g

- Fat: 7g

- Fiber: 4g

- Sugar: 18g

- Portion Size: 1 serving

Raspberry and Almond Butter Smoothie

Ingredients:

- 1 cup fresh raspberries
- 2 tablespoons almond butter
- 1/2 cup Greek yogurt
- 1 cup almond milk
- 1 tablespoon honey
- Ice cubes (optional)

Instructions:

1. Blend raspberries, almond butter, Greek yogurt, almond milk, and honey until well combined.
2. Add ice cubes if you prefer a chilled texture.
3. Pour into a glass and relish the delightful raspberry and almond fusion!

Nutrition Information (per serving):

- Calories: 220
- Protein: 7g
- Carbohydrates: 25g
- Fat: 10g

- Fiber: 8g

- Sugar: 15g

- Portion Size: 1 serving

Kiwi and Kale Immune Booster Smoothie

Ingredients:

- 2 kiwis, peeled and sliced

- 1 cup kale leaves, stems removed

- 1/2 cup pineapple chunks

- 1/2 lemon, juiced

- 1 tablespoon flaxseeds

- 1 cup coconut water

- Ice cubes (optional)

Instructions:

1. Blend kiwis, kale leaves, pineapple chunks, lemon juice, flaxseeds, and coconut water until smooth.

2. Add ice cubes if desired and blend again.

3. Pour into a glass and boost your immune system with this green elixir!

Nutrition Information (per serving):

- Calories: 100
- Protein: 3g
- Carbohydrates: 20g
- Fat: 2g
- Fiber: 5g
- Sugar: 10g
- Portion Size: 1 serving

Orange Creamsicle Smoothie

Ingredients:

- 1 cup fresh orange segments
- 1/2 cup vanilla Greek yogurt
- 1/2 cup almond milk
- 1 tablespoon honey
- 1/2 teaspoon vanilla extract
- Ice cubes (optional)

Instructions:

1. Blend orange segments, Greek yogurt, almond milk, honey, and vanilla extract until smooth.
2. Add ice cubes if you prefer a colder texture.

3. Pour into a glass and savor the nostalgic taste of an orange creamsicle!

Nutrition Information (per serving):

- Calories: 120
- Protein: 5g
- Carbohydrates: 25g
- Fat: 2g
- Fiber: 3g
- Sugar: 18g
- Portion Size: 1 serving

Mixed Berry Antioxidant Smoothie

Ingredients:

- 1/2 cup mixed berries (strawberries, blueberries, raspberries)
- 1/2 cup pomegranate seeds
- 1/2 banana
- 1/2 cup Greek yogurt
- 1 cup almond milk
- Ice cubes (optional)

Instructions:

1. Blend mixed berries, pomegranate seeds, banana, Greek yogurt, and almond milk until well combined.

2. Add ice cubes if you desire a chilled texture.

3. Pour into a glass and revel in the antioxidant-rich goodness of mixed berries!

Nutrition Information (per serving):

- Calories: 140
- Protein: 6g
- Carbohydrates: 25g
- Fat: 3g
- Fiber: 6g
- Sugar: 15g
- Portion Size: 1 serving

CONCLUSION

As we wrap up this journey through the pages of "Diabetic Cookbooks for Type 2 Diabetes Vegetarian," it's evident that crafting delectable meals for those managing diabetes doesn't mean compromising on taste or variety. This cookbook stands as a testament to the harmonious blend of health-conscious choices and the vibrant, rich world of vegetarian cuisine.

In our exploration, we've delved into the intricacies of managing type 2 diabetes with a vegetarian approach, emphasizing the importance of balanced nutrition and mindful meal planning. The 30-day meal plan serves not only as a practical guide but also as a transformative tool, offering a diverse range of dishes that go beyond mere sustenance.

From the energizing breakfasts that kickstart your day to the satisfying dinners that bring it to a close, each recipe has been thoughtfully curated to meet the unique dietary needs of individuals with type 2 diabetes. We've embraced the bounty of nature, incorporating whole grains, legumes, and an array of vegetables into every dish, ensuring a symphony of flavors with every bite.

The snacks and appetizers section proves that mindful munching can be both delightful and health-conscious, offering an assortment of treats to curb cravings without compromising on nutritional value. And as we dive into the sweet realm of desserts, we've demonstrated that indulgence can coexist with dietary restrictions through inventive recipes that celebrate natural sweetness and nourishing ingredients.

The refreshing smoothies provided in the final chapter are more than just beverages; they are a celebration of wholesome goodness, offering a burst of vitamins and antioxidants in every sip. These smoothies are a versatile addition to your daily routine, providing a tasty and nutritious option whether enjoyed as a snack, a meal replacement, or a post-workout refuel.

As you embark on your culinary journey with this cookbook, we encourage you to savor the joy of creating these dishes. It's not just about maintaining a diabetic-friendly diet; it's about relishing the artistry in the kitchen and the vibrancy that comes with every carefully chosen ingredient.

May this cookbook serve as a guide, a source of inspiration, and a companion on your path to wellness. Here's to the joy of savoring delicious, healthful meals that nourish both body and soul. Cheers to a vibrant life filled with flavorful choices!

www.ingramcontent.com/pod-product-compliance
Lightning Source LLC
Chambersburg PA
CBHW070949260726
48661CB00003B/1198